The Essential Keto Vegetarian Cookbook

Most Wanted Easy and Delicious Keto Vegetarian Recipes to Lose Weight Quickly

Lidia Wong

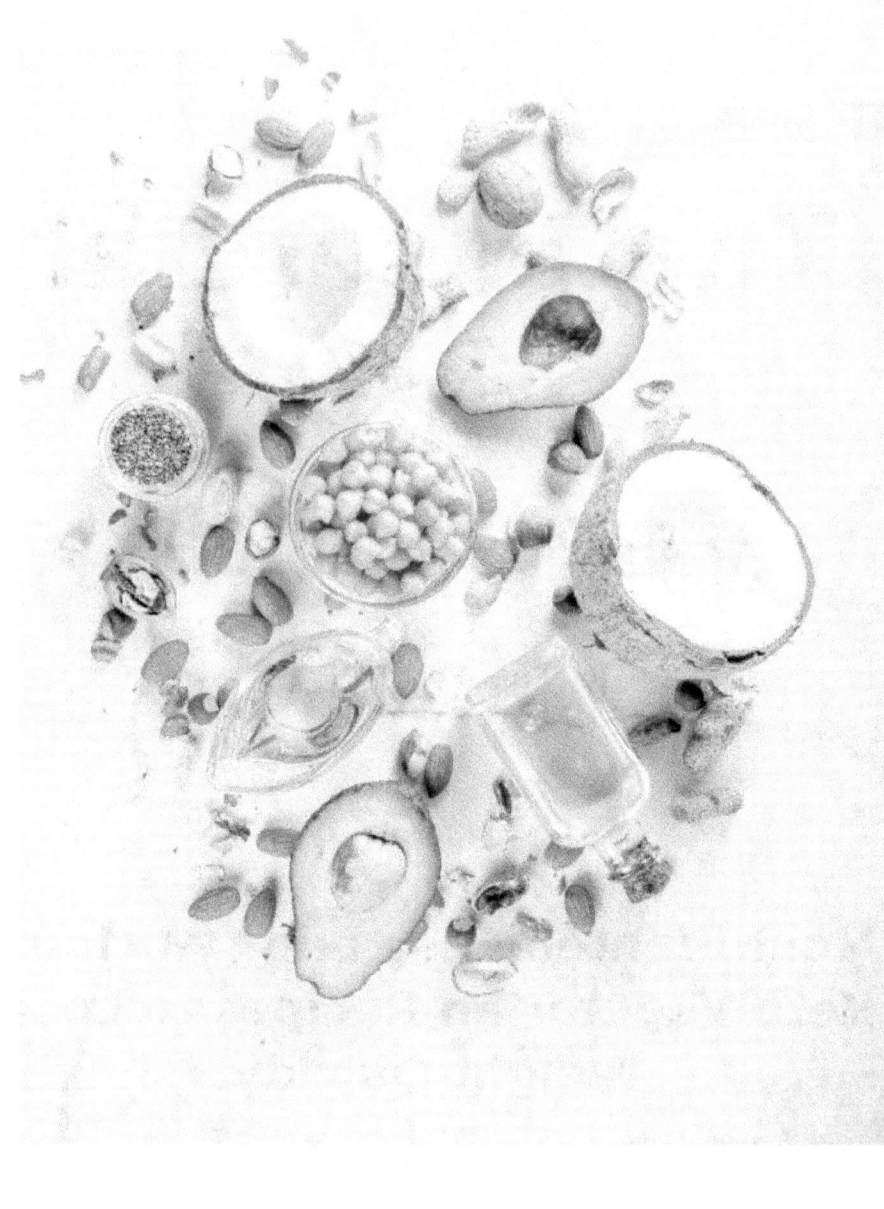

© **Copyright 2021 by Lidia Wong - All rights reserved.**

The content contained within this book may not be reproduced, duplicated or transmitted without direct written permission from the author or the publisher.
Under no circumstances will any blame or legal responsibility be held against the publisher, or author, for any damages, reparation, or monetary loss due to the information contained within this book. Either directly or indirectly.

Legal Notice:
This book is copyright protected. This book is only for personal use. You cannot amend, distribute, sell, use, quote or paraphrase any part, or the content within this book, without the consent of the author or publisher.

Disclaimer Notice:
Please note the information contained within this document is for educational and entertainment purposes only. All effort has been executed to present accurate, up to date, and reliable, complete information. No warranties of any kind are declared or implied. Readers acknowledge that the author is not engaging in the rendering of legal, financial, medical or professional advice. The content within this book has been derived from various sources. Please consult a licensed professional before attempting any techniques outlined in this book.
By reading this document, the reader agrees that under no circumstances is the author responsible for any losses, direct or indirect, which are incurred as a result of the use of information contained within this document, including, but not limited to, — errors, omissions, or inaccuracies.

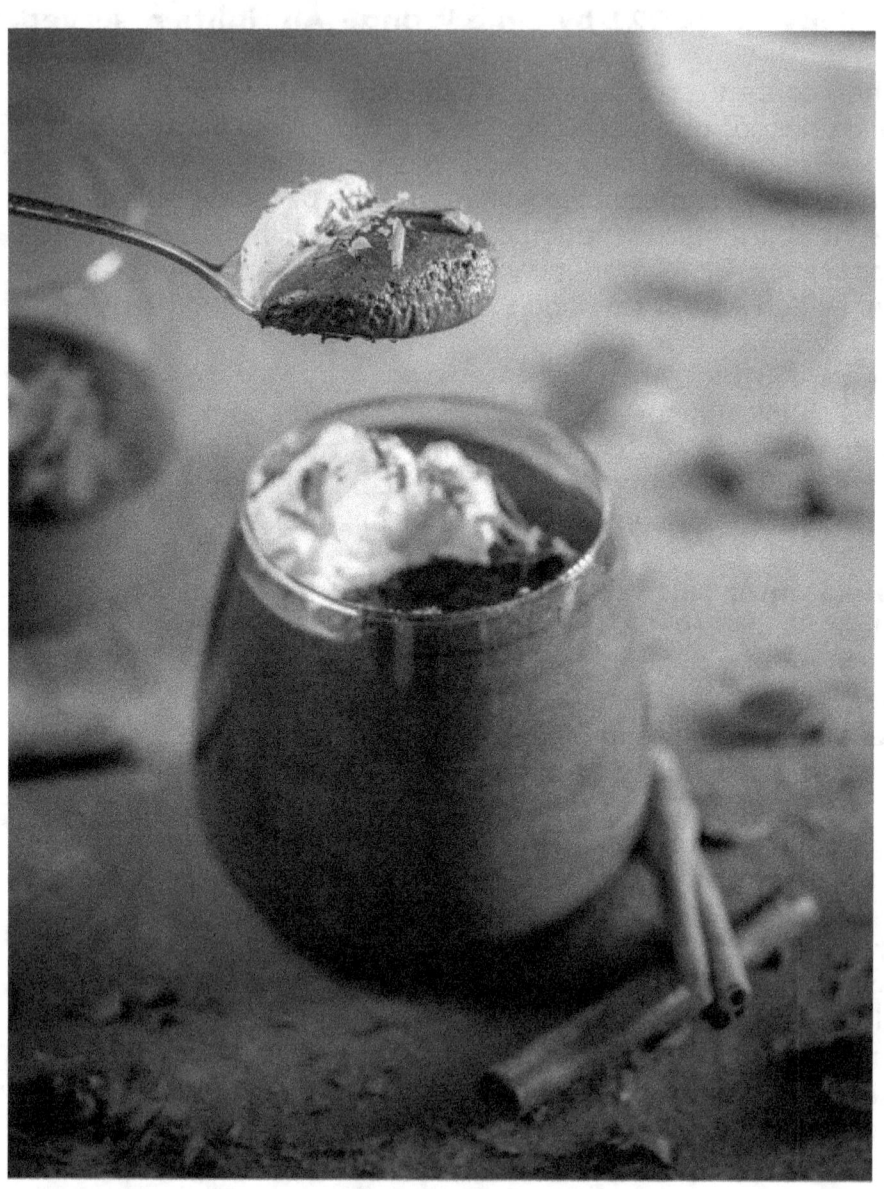

TABLE OF CONTENTS

INTRODUCTION 1

    Tomato and Avocado Pizza 3

    Creamy Cheese Soufflés.. 5

    Almond Flour Waffles 8

    Blueberry Chia Pudding 10

    Raspberry, Hazelnut and Pecan Porridge 12

    Curry Spinach Soup.. 14

    Zucchini and Cauliflower Soup 15

    Keto Caesar Salad 17

    Creamy Cabbage with Tofu and Pine Nuts................ 18

    Creamy Cajun Zucchinis... 20

    Oregano Zucchinis and Broccoli 21

    Garlic Asparagus and Tomatoes................................ 23

    Balsamic Hot Radishes.. 25

    Edamame Donburi 26

    Swiss Chard Salad 28

    Easy Corn Chowder 30

    Spinach, Tomato, and Orzo Soup 32

    Southern Succotash Stew 34

- Black Bean And Corn Soup 36
- Warm Vegetable "Salad" 38
- Golden Couscous Salad 40
- Ruby Grapefruit and Radicchio Salad 42
- Sunshine Fiesta Salad 44
- French-Style Potato Salad 46
- Roasted Carrot Salad 48
- Apple, Pecan, and Arugula Salad 50
- Caesar Salad 52
- Tempeh-Pimiento Cheese Ball 54
- Basil Rice Bowls 56
- Keto Hot Peppers C.s 58
- Light Cabbage Mayo Salad 60
- Zucchini and Amaranth Patties 61
- Cinnamon Coconut Chips 63
- Vegan Gumbo 64
- Feta Cheese (vegan) 66
- Truffle Parmesan Cheese (vegan) 68
- Eggplant Noodles with Sesame Tofu 71
- Rutabaga Hash Browns 75
- Crispy Flaxseed Waffles (ovo) 77
- Baked Cauliflower 80

Cabbage Cucumber Salad 82

Cashew-Chocolate Truffles 84

Fruits Stew 86

Mint Chocolate Cream 87

Cranberries Cake 88

Custard Bread Pudding 90

Low-Carb Curd Soufflé 92

Baked Rhubarb 93

Avocado Cupcakes 95

Rhubarb and Berries Cream 97

Chia Bowls 98

Almond Butter Brownies 99

NOTE **101**

INTRODUCTION

The keto diet is the shortened term for ketogenic diet and it is essentially a high-fat and low-carb diet that helps you lose weight, thereby bringing various health benefits. This diet drastically restricts your carb intake while increasing your fat intake; this pushes your body to go into a state know as "*ketosis*". We will tackle ketosis in a bit.

The human body uses glucose from carbs to fuel metabolic pathways—meaning various bodily functions like digestion, breathing, etc.. Essentially, anything that needs energy. Even when you are resting, the body needs fuel or energy for you to continue living. If you think about it, when have you ever stopped breathing, or your heart stopped beating, or your liver stopped from cleansing the body, or your kidneys from filtering blood?

Never, unless you're dead, which is the only time in which the body doesn't need energy. In normal circumstances, glucose is the primary pathway when it comes to sourcing the body's energy.

But the body also has another pathway; it can utilize fats to fuel the various bodily processes. And this is what we call "*ketosis*". And the body can only enter ketosis when there is no glucose available, thus the reason for sticking to a low-carb diet is essential in the keto diet. Since no glucose is available, the body is pushed to use fats—it can either come from the food you consume or from your body's fat reserves—the adipose tissue or from the flabby parts of your body. This is how the keto diet helps you lose weight, by burning up all those stored fats that you have and using it to fuel bodily processes.

That said, if for whatever reason you are a vegetarian, following a ketogenic diet can be extremely difficult. A vegetarian diet is largely free of animal products, which means that food tends to be usually high in carbohydrates. Still, with careful planning, it is possible. This Cookbook will provide you with various easy and delicious dishes to help you stick to your ketogenic diet plan while being a vegetarian.

Enjoy!

Tomato and Avocado Pizza

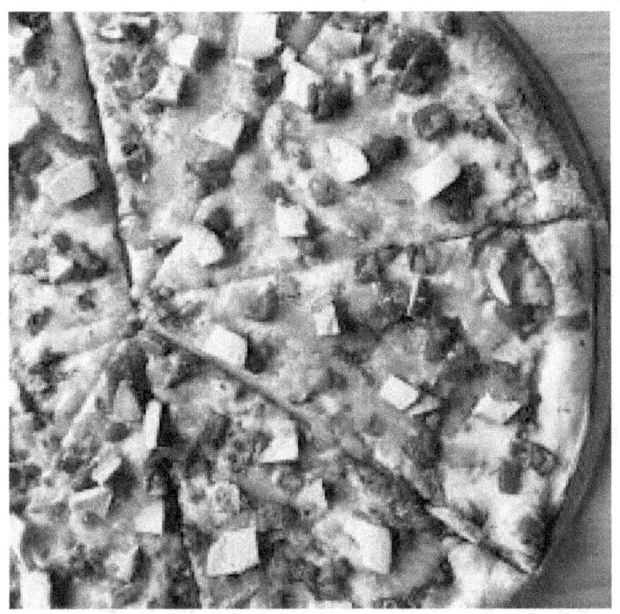

Preparation time: 20 minutes

Cooking time: 20 minutes

Servings: 2

Ingredients:

- 2 cups almond flour
- 1 avocado, peeled, pitted and sliced
- 1 and ½ cups water
- 2 tablespoons avocado oil

- 1 teaspoon chili powder
- 1 tomato, sliced
- A pinch of salt and black pepper
- ¼ cup tomato passata
- 2 tablespoons chives, chopped

Directions:

1. In a bowl, mix the flour with salt, pepper, water, oil and chili powder, stir well until you obtain a dough, knead a bit, put in a bowl, cover and leave aside for 20 minutes.
2. Transfer the dough to a working surface, shape a circle, transfer it to a baking sheet lined with parchment paper and bake at 400 degrees F for 10 minutes.
3. Spread the tomato passata over the pizza crust, also add the rest of the ingredients and bake at 400 degrees F for 10 minutes more.
4. Cut and serve for breakfast.

Nutrition:

calories 416, fat 24.5, fiber 9.6, carbs 36.6, protein 15.4

Creamy Cheese Soufflés

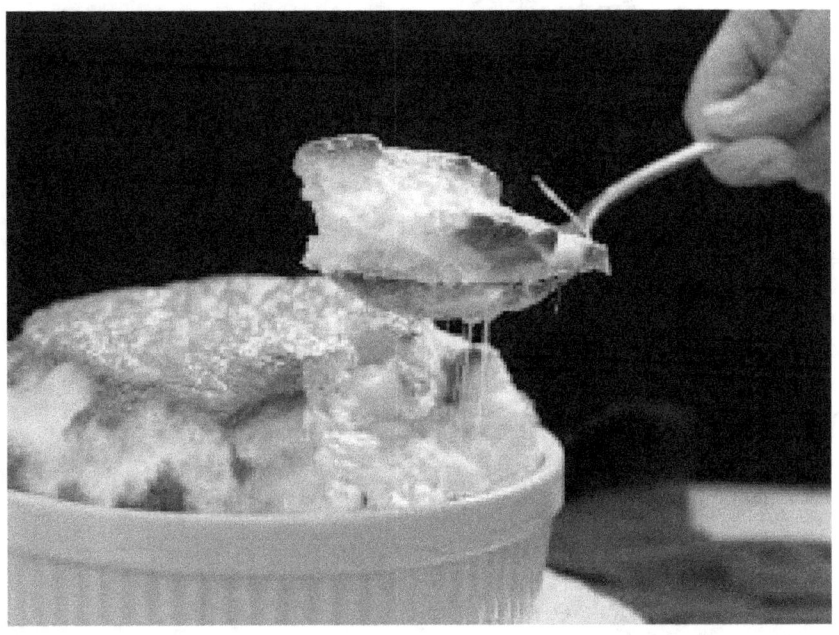

Preparation Time: 10 minutes

Cooking Time: 25 minutes

Servings: 8

Ingredients:

- 6 organic eggs, separated
- ½ cup almond flour
- 1 teaspoon salt

- ¾ cup heavy cream
- 1 teaspoon mustard, ground
- ½ teaspoon pepper
- ½ teaspoon xanthan gum
- ¼ teaspoon cayenne pepper
- 2 cups cheddar cheese, shredded
- 4 tablespoons chives, fresh, chopped
- ¼ teaspoon cream of tartar

Directions:

1. Preheat your oven to 350°Fahrenheit. Spray 8 ramekins with cooking spray and place them onto a cookie sheet.
2. In a mixing bowl, whisk together pepper, mustard, cayenne, xanthan gum, salt and almond flour.
3. Slowly add in the cream and mix until well combined.
4. Whisk your egg yolks, cheese, chives until well blended. In another mixing bowl, beat the egg whites with the cream of tartar until stiff peaks are formed.

5. Gently fold egg whites into the cheese and almond flour mixture. Pour the mixture into prepared ramekins.
6. Bake in preheated oven for 25 minutes or until your soufflés are lightly golden brown.
7. Serve and enjoy!

Nutritional Values (Per Serving):

Calories: 214 Fat: 17.9 g Carbohydrates: 1.6 g Sugar: 0.5 g Protein: 11.6 g Cholesterol: 168 mg

Almond Flour Waffles

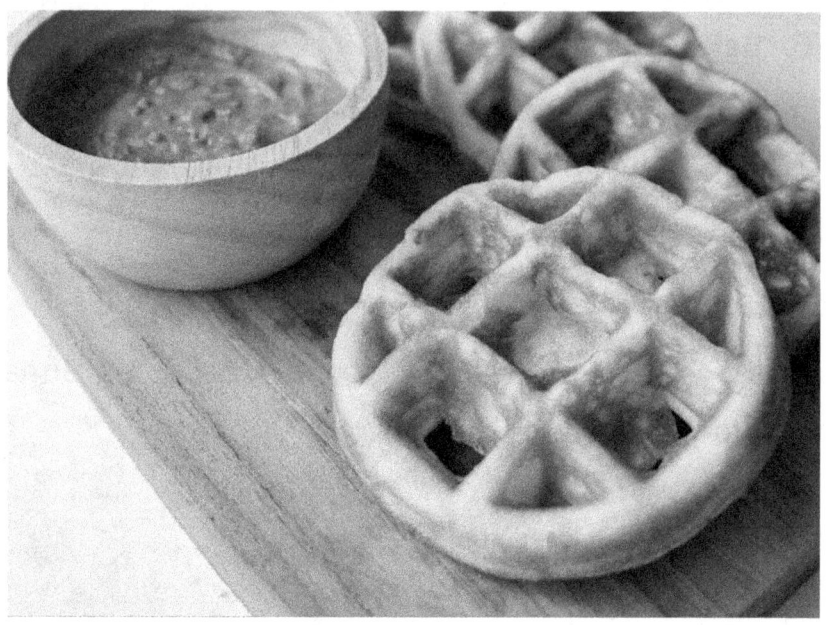

Preparation Time: 10 minutes

Cooking Time: 5 minutes

Servings: 2

Ingredients:

- 1 tablespoon butter, melted
- 1 large organic egg
- 2 tablespoons sour cream
- Pinch of xanthan gum

- Pinch of salt
- 1 teaspoon vinegar
- 2 teaspoons arrowroot flour
- 1/8 teaspoon baking powder
- 1/8 teaspoon baking soda
- ¼ cup almond flour

Directions:

1. In a mixing bowl combine vinegar, butter, sour cream, and egg mix well.
2. Add dry ingredients into wet and mix until well blended.
3. Heat your waffle iron and cook waffle for 5 minutes or to your waffle iron instructions.
4. Serve and enjoy!

Nutritional Values (Per Serving):

Calories: 208 Fat: 18 g Carbohydrates: 4.83 g Sugar: 2.1 g Protein: 6.52 g Cholesterol: 114 mg

Blueberry Chia Pudding

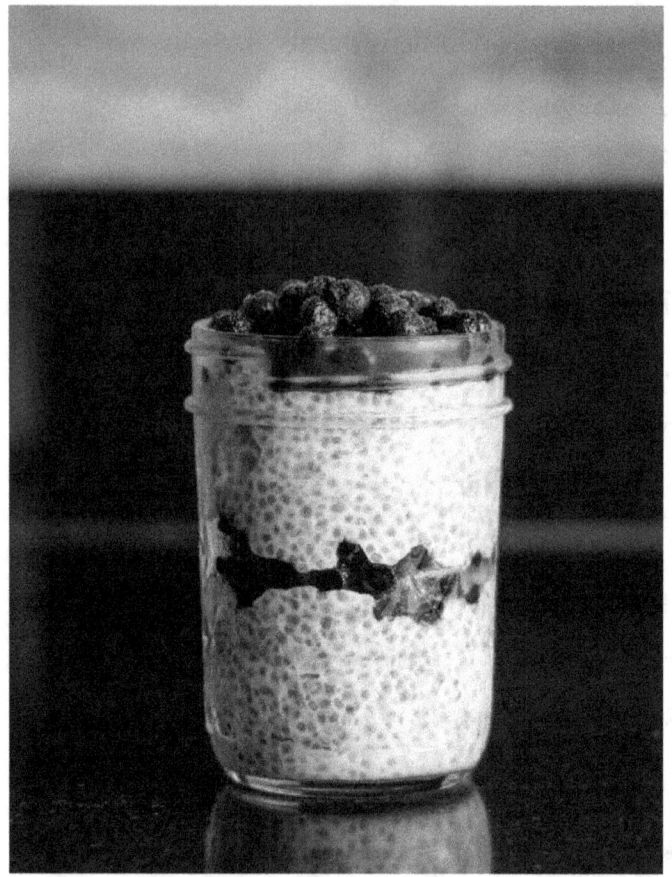

Preparation Time: 3 minutes + 4 hours refrigeration

Servings: 2

Ingredients:

- 2 tbsp chia seeds
- ¾ cup coconut milk
- ½ tsp vanilla extract
- ½ cup blueberries
- Chopped walnuts to garnish

Directions:

1. Mix all the ingredients in a medium bowl except for the walnuts.
2. Share the mixture into two breakfast jars, cover, and refrigerate for 4 hours or until the pudding gels.
3. Remove when ready to enjoy, top with some blueberries, walnuts, and serve immediately.

Nutrition:

Calories: 307, Total Fat:29.9 g, Saturated Fat:11.3 g, Total Carbs: 9 g, Dietary Fiber: 3g, Sugar: 4g, Protein:6 g, Sodium: 8mg

Raspberry, Hazelnut and Pecan Porridge

Preparation Time: 8 minutes

Cooking Time: 15 minutes

Serving: 2

Ingredients:

- 2 eggs
- 2 tbsp coconut flour
- 1 tsp psyllium husk powder
- 6 tbsp coconut cream
- 2 oz butter
- 2 tbsp chopped pecans
- 2 tbsp freshly squeezed lemon juice
- 1 tsp cinnamon powder
- 6 fresh raspberries, halved
- 4 tbsp chopped hazelnuts
- Salt to taste

Directions:

1. In a medium saucepan, combine the coconut flour, psyllium husk powder, salt, coconut cream, egg, lemon juice, and cinnamon powder.

2. Cook the ingredients over low heat while stirring constantly but do not allow boiling until thickened.
3. Dish the porridge and top with the raspberries, hazelnuts, and pecans.
4. Serve warm.

Nutrition:

Calories: 96, Total Fat: 9.9g, Saturated Fat:6.7 g, Total Carbs: 2 g, Dietary Fiber: 1, Sugar: 1g, Protein: 1g, Sodium: 66mg

Curry Spinach Soup

Preparation time: 10 minutes

Cooking time: 0 minutes

Servings: 4

Ingredients:

- 1 cup almond milk
- 1 tablespoon green curry paste
- 1 pound spinach leaves
- 1 tablespoon cilantro, chopped
- 4 cups veggie stock
- Salt and black pepper to the taste
- 1 tablespoon cilantro, chopped

Directions:

1. In your blender, combine the almond milk with the curry paste and the other ingredients, pulse well, divide into bowls and serve for lunch.

Nutrition:

calories 240, fat 4, fiber 2, carbs 6, protein 2

Zucchini and Cauliflower Soup

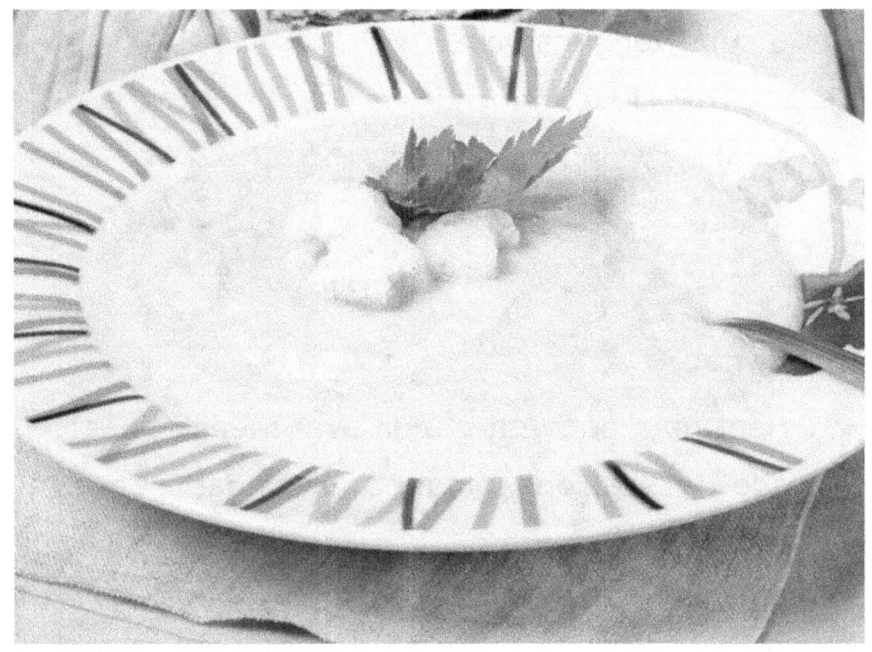

Preparation time: 10 minutes

Cooking time: 25 minutes

Servings: 4

Ingredients:

- 4 scallions, chopped
- 1 teaspoon ginger, grated
- 1 pound zucchinis, sliced

- 2 cups cauliflower florets
- Salt and black pepper to the taste
- 2 tablespoons olive oil
- 6 cups veggie stock
- 1 garlic clove, minced
- 1 tablespoon lemon juice
- 1 cup coconut cream

Directions:

1. Heat up a pot with the oil over medium heat, add the scallions, ginger and the garlic and sauté for 5 minutes.
2. Add the rest of the ingredients, bring to a simmer and cook over medium heat for 20 minutes.
3. Blend everything using an immersion blender, ladle into soup bowls and serve.

Nutrition:

calories 154, fat 12, fiber 3, carbs 5, protein 4

Keto Caesar Salad

Preparation Time: 15 minutes

Servings: 8

Ingredients:

- 8 cups romaine lettuce, chopped
- ¼ cup Parmesan cheese, grated, fresh
- 2 tablespoons lemon juice, fresh
- ¼ teaspoon garlic powder
- 1 tablespoon mayonnaise
- ¼ cup extra-virgin olive oil
- ¼ teaspoon pepper

Directions:

1. In a mixing bowl, combine olive oil, garlic powder, lemon juice and mayonnaise.
2. Add lettuce and cheese to the bowl. Season with pepper.
3. Cover bowl and place in the fridge for about an hour. Just before serving toss salad and enjoy!

Nutritional Values (Per Serving):

Calories: 102 Fat: 9.3 g Sugar: 0.8 g Cholesterol: 5 mg Carbohydrates: 2.3 g Protein: 3.3 g

Creamy Cabbage with Tofu and Pine Nuts

Preparation Time: 5 minutes

Cooking Time: 20 minutes

Serving: 4

Ingredients:

For the fried tofu:

- 25 oz tofu, cut into 6 slabs
- 2 tbsp butter

For the creamy cabbage:

- 2 oz butter
- 25 oz green canon cabbage, shredded
- 1 ¼ cups heavy cream
- Salt and black pepper to taste
- ½ cup chopped fresh marjoram
- ½ lemon, zested
- 2 tbsp toasted pine nuts

Directions:

For the fried tofu:

1. Melt the butter in a medium skillet over medium heat and fry the tofu on both sides until lightly brown on the outside, 10 minutes. Transfer to a plate and keep warm until ready to serve.

For the creamy cabbage:

2. Melt the butter in the skillet and sauté the cabbage while occasionally stirring until the cabbage turns golden brown, 4 minutes.
3. Mix in the heavy cream, allow bubbling, and season with the marjoram, salt, black pepper, and lemon zest.
4. Divide the tofu onto four plates, spoon the cabbage to the side of the tofu, and sprinkle the pine nuts on the cabbage.
5. Serve warm.

Nutrition:

Calories: 269, Total Fat: 21.6g, Saturated Fat: 7.8g, Total Carbs: 6g, Dietary Fiber: 1g, Sugar: 3g, Protein: 13g, Sodium: 298mg

Creamy Cajun Zucchinis

Preparation time: 10 minutes

Cooking time: 20 minutes

Servings: 4

Ingredients:

- 1 pound zucchinis, roughly cubed
- 2 tablespoons olive oil
- 4 scallions, chopped
- 1 teaspoon Cajun seasoning
- Salt and black pepper to the taste
- A pinch of cayenne pepper
- 1 cup coconut cream
- 1 tablespoon dill, chopped

Directions:

1. Heat up a pan with the oil over medium heat, add the scallions, cayenne and Cajun seasoning, stir and sauté for 5 minutes.
2. Add the zucchinis and the other ingredients, toss, cook over medium heat for 15 minutes more, divide between plates and serve.

Nutrition:

calories 200, fat 2, fiber 1, carbs 5, protein 8

Oregano Zucchinis and Broccoli

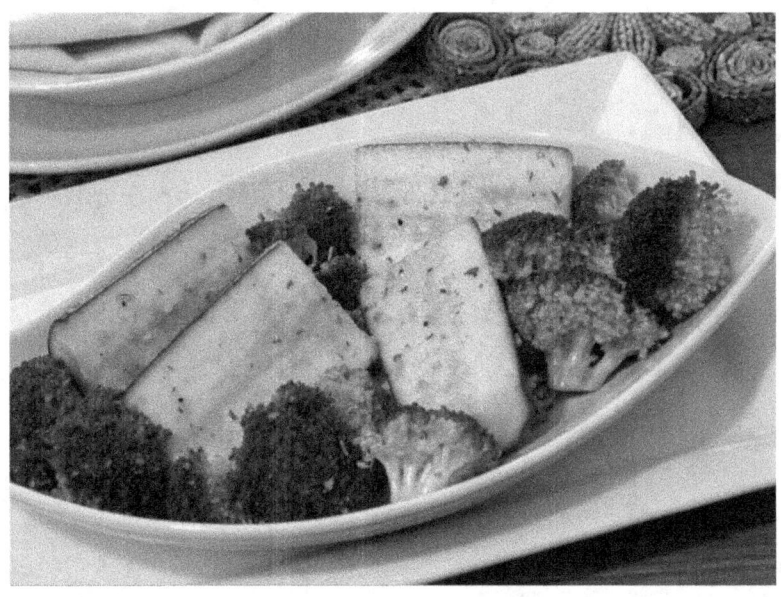

Preparation time: 10 minutes

Cooking time: 20 minutes

Servings: 4

Ingredients:

- 1 pound zucchinis, sliced
- 1 cup broccoli florets
- 2 tablespoons avocado oil
- Salt and black pepper to the taste

- 2 tablespoons chili powder
- ½ teaspoon oregano, dried
- 1 and ½ tablespoons coriander, chopped

Directions:

1. Heat up a pan with the oil over medium heat, add the zucchinis, broccoli and the other ingredients, toss, cook over medium heat for 20 minutes, divide between plates and serve as a side dish.

Nutrition:

calories 140, fat 2, fiber 1, carbs 1, protein 6

Garlic Asparagus and Tomatoes

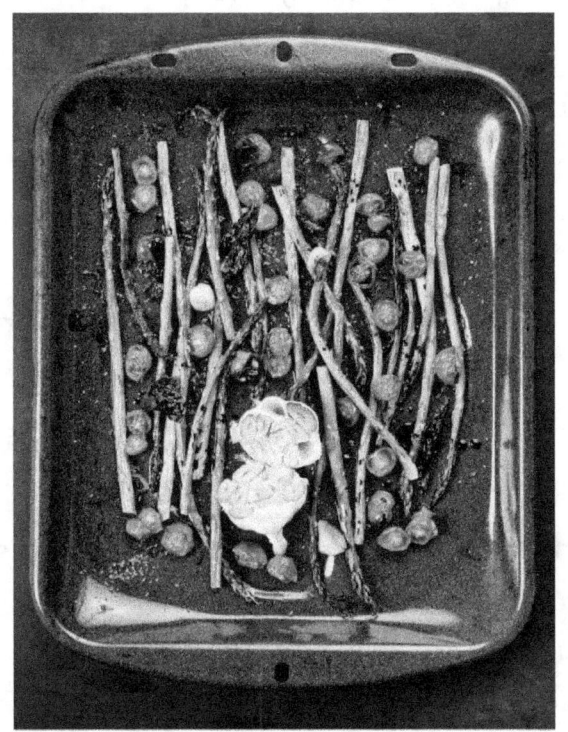

Preparation time: 10 minutes

Cooking time: 20 minutes

Servings: 4

Ingredients:

- 1 pound asparagus, trimmed and halved
- ½ pound cherry tomatoes, halved

- 1 teaspoon turmeric powder
- 2 tablespoons olive oil
- 2 tablespoons shallot, chopped
- A pinch of salt and black pepper
- 1 tablespoon chives, chopped

Directions:

1. Spread the asparagus on a baking sheet lined with parchment paper, add the tomatoes and the other ingredients, toss, cook in the oven at 375 degrees F for 20 minutes.
2. Divide everything between plates and serve as a side dish.

Nutrition:

calories 132, fat 1, fiber 2, carbs 4, protein 4

Balsamic Hot Radishes

Preparation time: 10 minutes

Cooking time: 20 minutes

Servings: 4

Ingredients:

- 2 tablespoons avocado oil
- 1 tablespoon balsamic vinegar
- 1 pound radishes, halved
- A pinch of salt and black pepper
- A pinch of chili powder

Directions:

1. Heat up a pan with the oil over medium heat, add the radishes, vinegar and the other ingredients, toss, cook for 20 minutes, divide between plates and serve as a side dish.

Nutrition:

calories 182, fat 5, fiber 5, carbs 9, protein 9

Edamame Donburi

Preparation time: 5 minutes

cooking time: 20 minutes

servings: 4

Ingredients

- 1 cup fresh or frozen shelled edamame
- 1 tablespoon canola or grapeseed oil
- 5 shiitake mushroom caps, lightly rinsed, patted dry, and cut into 1/4-inch strips
- 1 medium yellow onion, minced
- 1 teaspoon grated fresh ginger
- 3 green onions, minced
- 8 ounces firm tofu, drained and crumbled
- 2 tablespoons soy sauce
- 1 tablespoon toasted sesame oil
- 3 cups hot cooked white or brown rice
- 1 tablespoon toasted sesame seeds, for garnish

Directions

1. In a small saucepan of boiling salted water, cook the edamame until tender, about 10 minutes.
2. Drain and set aside.
3. In a large skillet, heat the canola oil over medium heat.
4. Add the onion, cover, and cook until softened, about 5 minutes.
5. Add the mushrooms and cook, uncovered, 5 minutes longer.
6. Stir in the ginger and green onions.
7. Add the tofu and soy sauce and cook until heated through, stirring to combine well, about 5 minutes.
8. Stir in the cooked edamame and cook until heated through, about 5 minutes.
9. Divide the hot rice among 4 bowls, top each with the edamame and tofu mixture, and drizzle on the sesame oil.
10. Sprinkle with sesame seeds and serve immediately.

Swiss Chard Salad

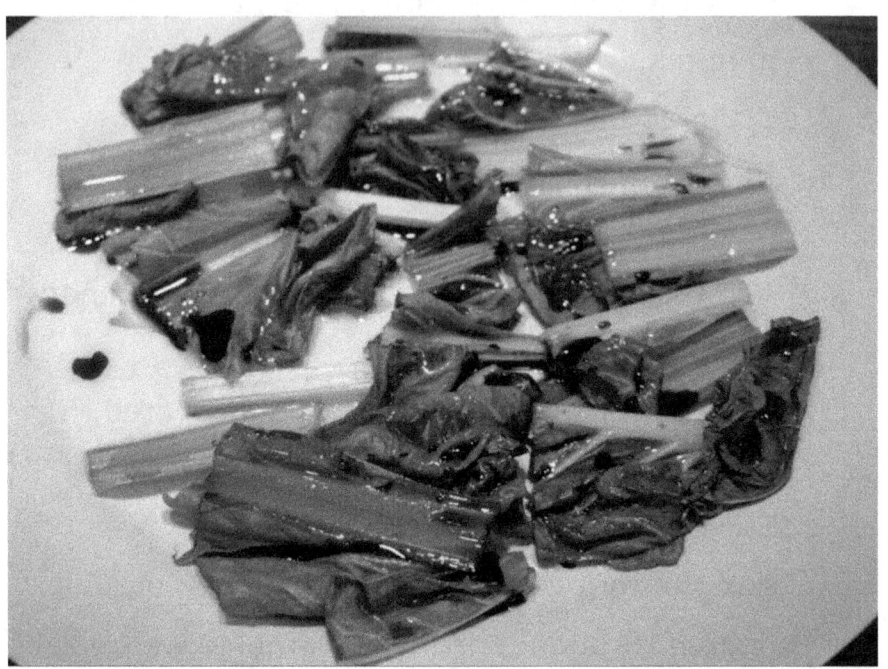

Preparation time: 10 minutes

Cooking time: 20 minutes

Servings: 4

Ingredients:

- 1 bunch Swiss chard, cut into strips
- 1 onion, peeled and chopped
- 2 tablespoons avocado oil

- A pinch of red pepper flakes
- ¼ cup pine nuts, toasted
- ¼ cup raisins
- 1 tablespoon balsamic vinegar
- Salt and ground black pepper, to taste

Directions:

1. Heat up a pan with the oil over medium heat, add the chard and onions, stir, and cook for 5 minutes.
2. Add the salt, pepper, and pepper flakes, stir, and cook for 3 minutes.
3. Put the raisins in a bowl, add the water to cover them, heat them up in a microwave for 1 minute, set aside for 5 minutes, and drain them well.
4. Add the raisins, and pine nuts to the pan with the vinegar, stir, cook for 3 minutes, divide on plates, and serve.

Nutrition:

Calories - 120, Fat - 2, Fiber - 1, Carbs - 4, Protein - 8

Easy Corn Chowder

Preparation time: 15 minutes

cooking time: 15 minutes

servings: 4

Ingredients

- 2 tablespoons olive oil or other vegetable oil, such as coconut oil
- 1 onion, chopped
- 1 cup chopped fennel bulb or celery
- 2 carrots, peeled and chopped
- 1 red bell pepper, finely chopped
- ¼ cup all-purpose flour
- 2 cups fresh or canned corn
- 6 cups vegetable stock
- 2 cups cubed red potato
- 1 cup unsweetened almond milk or other unsweetened nut or grain milk
- ½ teaspoon sriracha sauce or chili paste (optional)
- sea salt
- freshly ground black pepper

Directions

1. In a large pot, heat the olive oil over medium-high heat until it shimmers.
2. Add the onion, fennel, carrots, and bell pepper and cook, occasionally stirring, until the vegetables soften, about 3 minutes.
3. Sprinkle the flour over the vegetables and continue to cook, constantly stirring, for about 2 minutes.
4. Stir in the vegetable stock, using a spoon to scrape any bits of flour or vegetables from the bottom of the pan.
5. Continue stirring until the liquid comes to a boil and the soup begins to thicken. Lower the heat to medium.
6. Add the corn, potatoes, almond milk, and Sriracha, if using. Simmer until the potatoes are soft, about 10 minutes. Season with salt and pepper.
7. Serve hot.

Spinach, Tomato, and Orzo Soup

Preparation Time: 10 Minutes

Cooking Time: 20 Minutes

Servings: 6

Ingredients

- 1 tablespoon olive oil
- 1 onion, chopped
- 4 garlic cloves, minced
- 1 (14.5-ounce) can diced Italian tomatoes (preferably with oregano and basil)
- 4 cups water
- 4 cups low-sodium vegetable broth
- 1 teaspoon sea salt
- 1 teaspoon black pepper
- 1 pound uncooked orzo pasta
- 1 (5-ounce) package baby spinach

Directions

1. Preparing the ingredients
2. Heat the oil in a large stockpot over medium heat. Add the onion and sauté for 3 minutes, or

until soft. Add the garlic and sauté for 1 additional minute, or until fragrant.
3. Add the tomatoes with their juice, broth, water, salt, and pepper.
4. Cover the pot and bring to a boil.
5. Reduce the heat to a simmer.
6. Add the orzo and cook, uncovered, for 9 minutes, or until the pasta is tender.
7. Turn off the heat and stir in the spinach until wilted.

Southern Succotash Stew

Preparation Time: 5 Minutes

Cooking Time: 60 Minutes

Servings:4

Ingredients

- 8 ounces tempeh
- 2 tablespoons olive oil
- 1 large sweet yellow onion, finely chopped
- 2 carrots, cut into 1/4-inch slices
- 1 (14.5-ounce) can diced tomatoes, drained
- 2 medium russet potatoes, peeled and cut into 1/2-inch dice
- 1 (16-ounce) package frozen succotash
- 2 cups vegetable broth or water
- 1/2 teaspoon dried thyme
- 1/2 teaspoon ground allspice
- 2 tablespoons soy sauce
- 1 teaspoon dry mustard
- 1/4 teaspoon ground cayenne
- Salt and freshly ground black pepper
- 1/2 teaspoon liquid smoke

Directions

1. In a medium saucepan of simmering water, cook the tempeh for 30 minutes. Drain, pat dry, and cut into 1-inch dice.
2. In a large skillet, heat 1 tablespoon of the oil over medium heat. Add the tempeh and cook until browned on both sides, about 10 minutes. Set aside.
3. In a large saucepan, heat the remaining 1 tablespoon oil over medium heat. Add the onion and cook until softened, 5 minutes. Add the potatoes, carrots, tomatoes, succotash, broth, soy sauce, mustard, sugar, thyme, allspice, and cayenne. Season with salt and pepper to taste. Bring to a boil, then reduce heat to low and add the tempeh. Simmer, covered, until the vegetables are tender, occasionally stirring, about 45 minutes.
4. About 10 minutes before the stew is finished cooking, stir in the liquid smoke. Taste, adjusting seasonings if necessary. Serve immediately.

Black Bean And Corn Soup

Preparation Time: 5 Minutes

Cooking Time: 50 Minutes

Servings: 4

Ingredients

- 2 tablespoons olive oil
- 1 medium red onion, chopped
- 1 medium red or yellow bell pepper, chopped
- 1 medium carrot, minced
- 1 teaspoon ground cumin
- 4 garlic cloves, minced
- 1 teaspoon dried oregano
- 1 (14.5-ounce) can diced tomatoes, drained
- 4 1/2 cups cooked or 3 (15.5-ounce) cans black beans, rinsed and drained
- 6 cups vegetable broth, homemade (see Light Vegetable Broth) or store-bought, or water
- 2 cups fresh, frozen, or canned corn kernels
- 1 teaspoon fresh lemon juice
- Salt and freshly ground black pepper
- Tabasco sauce, to serve

Directions

1. In a large soup pot, heat the oil over medium heat. Add the onion, bell pepper, carrot, and garlic, cover, and cook until soft, about 10 minutes.
2. Uncover and stir in the cumin and oregano, tomatoes, beans, and broth. Bring to a boil, then reduce heat to low and simmer, uncovered, for 30 minutes, stirring occasionally.
3. Puree about one-third of the soup in the pot with an immersion blender, or in a blender or food processor, then return to the pot.
4. Add the corn, and simmer uncovered, for 10 minutes to heat through and blend flavors.
5. Just before serving, stir in the lemon juice and season with salt and pepper to taste.
6. Ladle into bowls and serve with hot sauce on the side.

Warm Vegetable "Salad"

Preparation time: 10 minutes

cooking time: 15 minutes

servings: 4

Ingredients

- 4 red potatoes, quartered
- 1 pound carrots, sliced into ¼-inch-thick rounds
- 1 tablespoon extra-virgin olive oil (optional)
- 2 tablespoons lime juice
- Salt for salting water, plus ½ teaspoon (optional)
- 2 teaspoons dried dill
- ¼ teaspoon freshly ground black pepper
- 1 cup Cashew Cream or Parm-y Kale Pesto

Directions

1. In a large pot, bring salted water to a boil. Add the potatoes and cook for 8 minutes.
2. Add the carrots and continue to boil for another 8 minutes, until both the potatoes and carrots are crisp tender.

3. Drain and return to the pot.
4. Add the olive oil (if using), lime juice, dill, remaining ½ teaspoon of salt (if using), and pepper, and stir to coat well.
5. Divide the vegetables evenly among 4 single-compartment storage containers or wide-mouth pint glass jars, and spoon ¼ cup of cream or pesto over the vegetables in each.
6. Let cool before sealing the lids.

Nutrition:

Calories: 393; Fat: 15g; Protein: 10g; Carbohydrates: 52g; Fiber: 9g; Sugar: 8g; Sodium: 343mg

Golden Couscous Salad

Preparation time: 5 minutes

cooking time: 12 minutes

servings: 4

Ingredients

- 1 cup couscous
- 1/4 cup olive oil
- 1 medium shallot, minced
- 1 medium yellow bell pepper, chopped
- 1 medium carrot, shredded
- 1/2 teaspoon ground coriander
- 1/2 teaspoon turmeric
- 1/4 teaspoon ground cayenne
- 2 cups vegetable broth, homemade or store-bought, or water
- Salt
- 1/2 cup chopped dried apricots
- 1/4 cup golden raisins
- 1/4 cup chopped unsalted roasted cashews
- 11/2 cups cooked or 1 (15.5-ouncecan chickpeas, drained and rinsed
- 2 tablespoons minced fresh cilantro leaves

- 2 tablespoons fresh lemon juice

Directions

1. In a large saucepan, heat 1 tablespoon of the oil over medium heat. Add the shallot, coriander, turmeric, cayenne, and couscous and stir until fragrant, about 2 minutes, being careful not to burn.
2. Stir in the broth and salt to taste. Bring to a boil, then remove from the heat, cover, and let stand for 10 minutes.
3. Transfer the cooked couscous to a large bowl. Add the bell pepper, carrot, apricots, raisins, cashews, chickpeas, and cilantro. Toss gently to combine and set aside.
4. In a small bowl, combine the remaining 3 tablespoons of oil with the lemon juice, stirring to blend.
5. Pour the dressing over the salad, toss gently to combine, and serve.

Ruby Grapefruit and Radicchio Salad

Preparation Time: 10 Minutes

Cooking Time: 0 Minutes

Servings: 4

Ingredients

For The Salad

- 1 large ruby grapefruit
- 1 small head radicchio, torn into bite-size pieces
- 2 cups baby spinach
- 2 cups green leaf lettuce, torn into bite-size pieces
- 1 bunch watercress
- 4 to 6 radishes, sliced paper-thin

For The Dressing

- juice of 1 lemon
- 2 teaspoons agave
- 1 teaspoon white wine vinegar
- ½ teaspoon freshly ground black pepper
- ½ teaspoon sea salt
- ¼ cup extra-virgin olive oil

Directions

1. To make the salad: Cut both ends off of the grapefruit, stand it on a cutting board on one of the flat sides, and, using a sharp knife, cut away the peel and all of the white pith. Remove the individual segments by slicing between the membrane and fruit on each side of each segment, dropping the fruit into a large salad bowl as you go. Add the radicchio, lettuce, spinach, watercress, and radishes to the bowl and toss well.
2. To make the dressing: Whisk together the lemon juice, agave, vinegar, salt, and pepper. Slowly whisk in the olive oil until the mixture is well combined and -emulsified. Toss the salad with the dressing and serve immediately.

Sunshine Fiesta Salad

Preparation Time: 15 Minutes

Cooking Time: 0 Minutes

Servings: 4

Ingredients

For The Vinaigrette

- Juice of 2 limes
- 1 tablespoon olive oil
- 1 tablespoon maple syrup or agave
- ¼ teaspoon sea salt

For The Salad

- 2 cups cooked quinoa
- 2 heads romaine lettuce, roughly chopped
- 1 tablespoon Taco Seasoning or store-bought taco seasoning
- 1 (15-ounce) can black beans, rinsed and drained
- 1 cup cherry tomatoes, halved
- 1 cup frozen (and thawed) or fresh corn kernels
- 1 avocado, peeled, pitted, and diced
- 4 scallions, thinly sliced

- 12 tortilla chips, crushed

Directions

1. To make the vinaigrette: In a small bowl, whisk together all the vinaigrette ingredients.
2. To make the salad: In a medium bowl, mix together the quinoa and taco seasoning. In a large bowl, toss the romaine with the vinaigrette.
3. Divide among 4 bowls. Top each bowl with equal amounts quinoa, beans, tomatoes, corn, avocado, scallions, and crushed tortillas chips.

French-Style Potato Salad

Preparation Time: 5 Minutes

Cooking Time: 30 Minutes

Servings: 4 To 6

Ingredients

- 1 1/2 pounds small white potatoes, unpeeled
- 2 tablespoons minced fresh parsley
- 1 tablespoon minced fresh chives
- 1 teaspoon minced fresh tarragon or 1/2 teaspoon dried
- 1/8 teaspoon freshly ground black pepper
- 1/3 cup olive oil
- 2 tablespoons white wine or tarragon vinegar

Directions

1. In a large pot of boiling salted water, cook the potatoes until tender but still firm, about 30 minutes.
2. Drain and cut into 1/4-inch slices. Transfer to a large bowl and add the parsley, chives, and tarragon. Set aside.

3. In a small bowl, combine the oil, vinegar, pepper.
4. Pour the dressing onto the potato mixture and toss gently to combine.
5. Taste, adjusting seasonings if necessary.
6. Chill for 1 to 2 hours before serving.

Roasted Carrot Salad

Preparation Time: 10 Minutes

Cooking Time: 30 Minutes

Servings: 3

Ingredients

- 4 carrots, peeled and sliced
- 1 to 2 teaspoons olive oil or coconut oil
- ½ teaspoon ground cinnamon or pumpkin pie spice
- 1 (15-ounce) can cannellini beans or navy beans, drained and rinsed
- 3 cups chopped hearty greens, such as spinach, kale, chard, or collards
- ⅓ cup dried cranberries or pomegranate seeds
- ⅓ cup slivered almonds or Cinnamon-Lime Sunflower Seeds
- Salt
- ¼ cup Raspberry Vinaigrette or Cilantro-Lime Dressing, or 2 tablespoons freshly squeezed orange or lemon juice whisked with 2 tablespoons olive oil and a pinch of salt

Directions

1. Preheat the oven or toaster oven to 400 °F.
2. In a medium bowl, toss the carrots with the olive oil and cinnamon and season to taste with salt.
3. Transfer to a small tray, and roast for 15 minutes or until browned around the edges. Toss the carrots, add the beans, and roast for 15 minutes more.
4. Let cool while you prep the salad. Divide the greens among three plates or containers, top with the cranberries and almonds, and add the roasted carrots and beans.
5. Drizzle with the dressing of your choice.
6. Store leftovers in an airtight container in the refrigerator for up to 1 week.

Apple, Pecan, and Arugula Salad

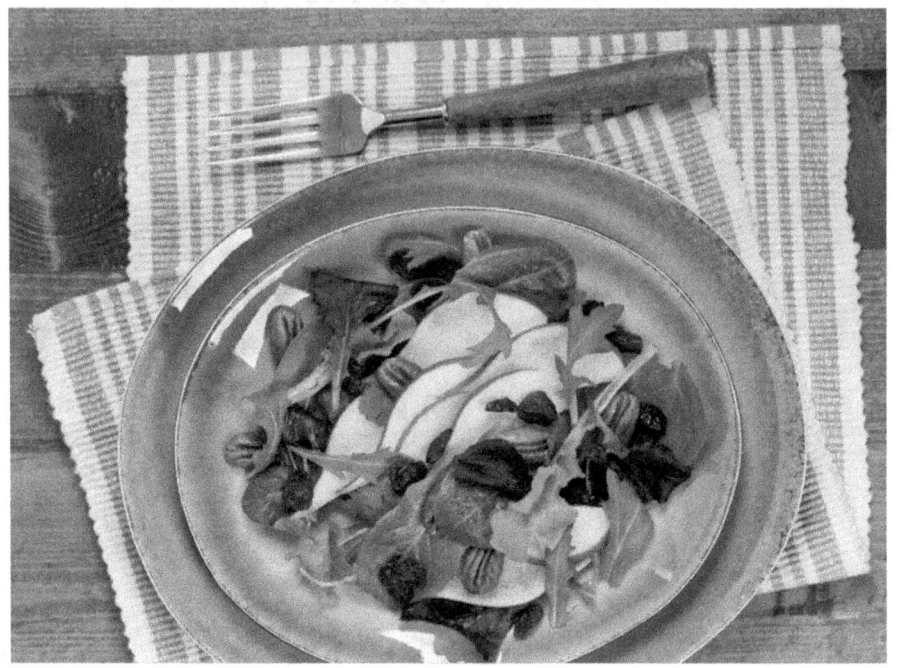

Preparation Time: 10 Minutes

Cooking Time: 0 Minutes

Servings: 4

Ingredients

- Juice of 1 lemon
- 2 tablespoons olive oil

- 1 tablespoon maple syrup
- 1 (5-ounce) package arugula
- 1 cup frozen (and thawed) or fresh corn kernels
- ½ red onion, thinly sliced
- 2 apples (preferably Gala or Fuji), cored and sliced
- 2 pinches sea salt
- ½ cup chopped pecans
- ¼ cup dried cranberries

Directions

1. In a small bowl, whisk together the lemon juice, oil, maple syrup, and salt.
2. In a large bowl, combine the arugula, corn, red onion, and apples.
3. Add the lemon juice mixture and toss to combine.
4. Divide evenly among 4 plates and top with the pecans and cranberries.

Caesar Salad

Preparation Time: 10 Minutes

Cooking Time: 0 Minutes

Servings: 1

Ingredients

For The Caesar Salad

- 2 cups chopped romaine lettuce
- 2 tablespoons Caesar Dressing
- 1 serving Herbed Croutons or store-bought croutons
- Vegan cheese, grated (optional)

Make It A Meal

- ½ cup cooked pasta
- ½ cup canned chickpeas, drained and rinsed
- 2 additional tablespoons Caesar Dressing

Directions

1. To Make The Caesar Salad. In a large bowl, toss together the lettuce, dressing, croutons, and cheese (if using).

2. To Make It A Meal. Add the pasta, chickpeas, and additional dressing. Toss to coat.

Nutrition Per Serving (in a meal)

Calories: 415; Protein: 19g; Total fat: 8g; Saturated fat: 1g; Carbohydrates: 72g; Fiber: 13g

Tempeh-Pimiento Cheese Ball

Preparation time: 5 minutes

cooking time: 30 minutes

servings: 8

Ingredients

- 8 ounces tempeh, cut into 1/2-inch pieces
- 1 (2-ouncejar chopped pimientos, drained
- 1/4 cup nutritional yeast
- 1/4 cup vegan mayonnaise, homemade or store-bought
- ¾ cup chopped pecans
- 2 tablespoons soy sauce

Directions

1. In a medium saucepan of simmering water, cook the tempeh for 30 minutes. Set aside to cool.
2. In a food processor, combine the cooled tempeh, pimientos, nutritional yeast, mayo, and soy sauce.
3. Process until smooth.

4. Transfer the tempeh mixture to a bowl and refrigerate until firm and chilled, at least 2 hours or overnight.
5. In a dry skillet, toast the pecans over medium heat until lightly toasted, about 5 minutes. Set aside to cool.
6. Shape the tempeh mixture into a ball, and roll it in the pecans, pressing the nuts slightly into the tempeh mixture so they stick.
7. Refrigerate for at least 1 hour before serving. If not using right away, cover and keep refrigerated until needed. Properly stored, it will keep for 2 to 3 days.

Basil Rice Bowls

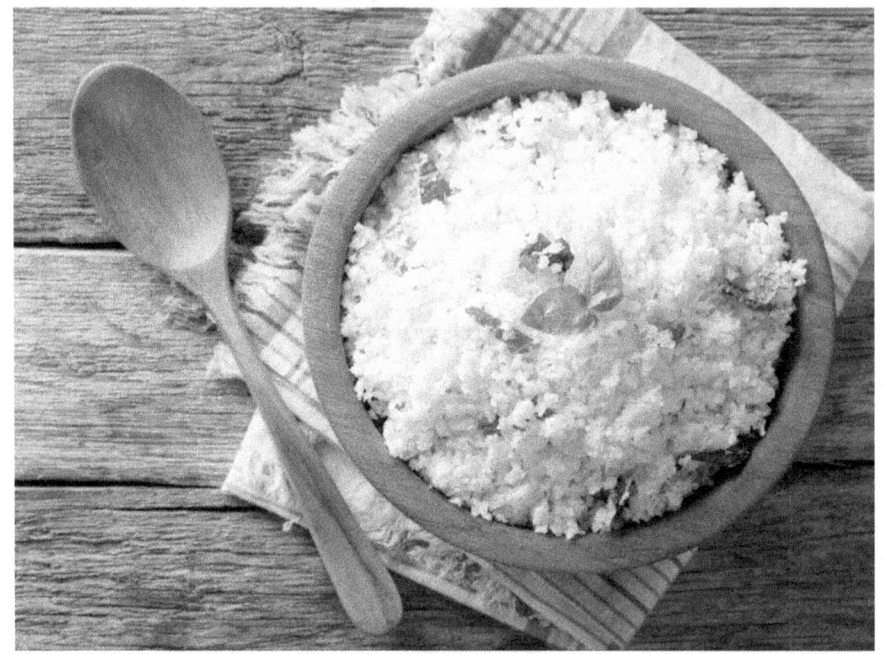

Preparation time: 10 minutes

Cooking time: 20 minutes

Servings: 4

Ingredients:

- 2 cups cauliflower rice
- 1 cup veggie stock
- 1 teaspoon turmeric powder

- 1 teaspoon cumin, ground
- 1 teaspoon fennel seeds, crushed
- 2 tablespoons olive oil
- 2 tomatoes, cubed
- 1 cup black olives, pitted and sliced
- 1 bunch basil, chopped
- A pinch of salt and black pepper

Directions:

1. Heat up a pan with the oil over medium heat, add the cauliflower rice, stock, salt, pepper and the other ingredients, stir, cook for 20 minutes, divide into small bowls and serve as an appetizer.

Nutrition:

calories 118, fat 11.5, fiber 2.2, carbs 5.9, protein 4

Keto Hot Peppers C.s

Preparation Time: 15 minutes

Cooking Time: 15-20 minutes

Servings: 4

Ingredients

- 4 eggs, beaten
- 3 hot red peppers, dried
- 4 freshly chopped basil leaves
- 8 tbsps. buckwheat flour
- 2 tsps. baking powder
- 2½ tbsps. coconut milk
- 1 tbsp. olive oil
- ½ tsp. salt

Directions:

1. Preheat oven to 380 °F.
2. In a bowl, mix the eggs, coconut milk, fresh basil and hot peppers.
3. In a separate mixing bowl, mix the buckwheat flour with the baking powder and salt.

4. Unite the egg mixture with the flour mixture and stir well.
5. Pour the batter in cups (3/4 c. full).
6. Bake in oven for 15-20 minutes.
7. When ready let cool and serve.

Nutrition:

Calories: 35, Fat: 11.65g, Carbs: 16.33g, Protein: 12.57g

Light Cabbage Mayo Salad

Preparation Time: 5 minutes

Cooking Time: 0 minutes

Servings: 2

Ingredients

- ½ medium cabbage head
- ¼ c. Mayonnaise gluten-free, grain free
- 2 tbsps. Cheddar cheese
- Salt

Directions:

1. Wash your cabbage and rinse. The outermost leaves should be removed.
2. Half the cabbage and chop.
3. Place the cabbage in large container and season with salt.
4. Pour mayonnaise and stir well.
5. You can refrigerate salad about one hour before serving.
6. Sprinkle with Cheddar cheese if used and serve.

Nutrition:

Calories: 99.59, Fat: 3.62g, Carbs: 6.86g, Protein: 5.33g

Zucchini and Amaranth Patties

Preparation Time: 10 minutes

Cooking Time: 30 minutes

Servings: 14

Ingredients:

- 1 1/2 cups shredded zucchini
- ½ of a medium onion, shredded
- 1 1/2 cups cooked white beans
- 1/2 cup amaranth seeds
- 1 teaspoon red chili powder
- 1/4 cup flax meal
- 1/2 teaspoon cumin
- 1/2 cup cornmeal
- 1 tablespoon salsa
- 1 1/2 cups vegetable broth

Directions:

1. Stir together stock and amaranth on a pot, bring it to a boil over medium-high heat, then switch heat to medium-low level and simmer until all the liquid is absorbed.

2. Mash the white beans in a bowl, add remaining ingredients, including cooked amaranth and stir until well mixed.
3. Shape the mixture into patties, then place them on a baking sheet lined with parchment sheet and bake for 30 minutes until browned and crispy, turning halfway.
4. Serve straight away.

Nutrition:

Calories:152 Cal, Fat: 3 g, Carbs: 29 g, Protein: 7 g, Fiber: 6 g

Cinnamon Coconut Chips

Preparation Time: 5 minutes

Cooking Time: 2 minutes

Servings: 2

Ingredients:

- ¼ cup coconut chips, unsweetened
- ¼ teaspoon sea salt
- ¼ cup cinnamon

Directions:

1. Add cinnamon and salt in a mixing bowl and set aside.
2. Heat a pan over medium heat for 2 minutes.
3. Place the coconut chips in the hot pan and stir until coconut chips crisp and lightly brown.
4. Toss toasted coconut chips with cinnamon and salt.
5. Serve and enjoy!

Nutrtions:

Calories: 228 Carbohydrates: 7.8 g Fat: 21 g Sugar: 0 g Cholesterol: 0 mg Protein: 1.9 g

Vegan Gumbo

Preparation time: 10 minutes

Cooking time: 8 hours

Servings: 4

Ingredients:

- 2 tablespoons olive oil
- 1 green bell pepper, chopped
- 1 yellow onion, chopped
- 15 ounces canned tomatoes, chopped
- 2 celery stalks, chopped
- 3 garlic cloves, minced
- 2 cups veggie stock
- 8 ounces white mushrooms, sliced
- 15 ounces canned kidney beans, drained
- 1 zucchini, chopped
- 1 tablespoon Cajun seasoning
- Salt and black pepper to the taste

Directions:

1. In your slow cooker, mix oil with bell pepper, onion, celery, garlic, tomatoes, stock,

mushrooms, beans, zucchini, Cajun seasoning, salt and pepper, stir, cover and cook on Low for 8 hours
2. Divide into bowls and serve hot.
3. Enjoy!

Nutritions:

calories 312, fat 4, fiber 7, carbs 19, protein 4

Feta Cheese (vegan)

Preparation time: 20 minutes

Cooking time: 0 minute

Servings: 4

Ingredients:

- 1 13-oz. block extra firm tofu (drained)
- 3 cups water
- ¼ cup apple cider vinegar
- 2 tbsp. dark miso paste
- 1 tbsp. sun dried tomatoes (chopped)
- 1 tsp. ground black pepper
- 2 garlic cloves
- 2 tsp. Himalayan salt

Directions:

1. Cut the tofu into ½-inch cubes and put them into a medium-sized saucepan with 2 cups of water.
2. Bring the water to a boil over medium-high heat, take the pan off the heat immediately, drain half of the water, and set aside to let it

cool down.

3. Pour the vinegar, miso paste, pepper, salt, and the remaining 1 cup of water into a blender or food processor. Blend until everything is well combined.
4. Pour the liquid from the blender into an airtight container. Add the garlic cloves, sundried tomatoes, and the tofu (including the water) to the container.
5. Give the feta cheese a good stir and then store in the fridge or freezer for at least 4 hours before serving.
6. Serve with low-carb crackers, or, enjoy this delicious feta cheese in a healthy salad!
7. Alternatively, store the cheese in an airtight container in the fridge and consume within 6 days. Store for a maximum of 30 days in the freezer and thaw at room temperature.

Nutritions:

Calories: 101kcal, Carbs: 5.2g, Net Carbs: 3.8g, Fat: 4.9g, Protein: 10.3g, Fiber:1.4g, Sugar: 0.7g

Truffle Parmesan Cheese (vegan)

Preparation time: 30 minutes

Cooking time: 0 minute

Servings: 8

Ingredients:

- 1 cup macadamia nuts (unsalted)
- 1 cup raw cashews (unsalted)
- 2 garlic cloves
- 2 tbsp. truffle oil
- ½ tbsp. nutritional yeast
- 1 tsp. agar-agar
- 1 tsp. fresh lime juice
- 1 tsp. dark miso paste

Directions:

1. Cover the cashews with water in a small bowl and let sit for 4 to 6 hours.
2. Rinse and drain the cashews after soaking. Make sure no water is left.

3. Preheat the oven to 350°F / 175°C, and line a baking sheet with parchment paper.
4. Put the macadamia nuts on a baking sheet and spread them out, so they can roast evenly.
5. Transfer the baking sheet to the oven and roast the macadamia nuts for about 8 minutes, until slightly browned.
6. Take the nuts out of the oven and set them aside, allowing them to cool down.
7. Grease a medium-sized shallow baking dish with ½ tablespoon of truffle oil.
8. Add the soaked cashews, roasted macadamia nuts, and all the remaining ingredients to a blender or food processor.
9. Blend everything into a crumbly mixture.
10. Transfer the crumbly parmesan into the baking dish, spread it out evenly, and firmly press it down until it has fused together into an even layer of cheese.
11. Cover the baking dish with aluminum foil and refrigerate the cheese for 8 hours or until the parmesan is firm.

12. Serve or store the cheese in an airtight container in the fridge and consume within 6 days.
13. Store for a maximum of 60 days in the freezer and thaw at room temperature.

Nutritions:

Calories: 202kcal, Net Carbs: 4.4g, Fat: 18.7g
Protein: 4g, Fiber: 1.8g, Sugar: 1.8g

Eggplant Noodles with Sesame Tofu

Preparation Time: 25 minutes

Cooking Time: 20-22 minutes

Servings: 4

Ingredients:

- 1 pound block firm tofu
- 1 cup chopped cilantro
- 3 tablespoons rice vinegar
- 2 cloves garlic, finely minced
- 4 tablespoons toasted sesame oil
- 1 teaspoon crushed red pepper flakes
- 2 teaspoons Swerve confectioners
- 1 whole eggplant
- 1 tablespoon olive oil
- Salt and pepper to taste
- ¼ cup sesame seeds
- ¼ cup soy sauce

Directions:

1. Preheat oven to 200 °F.
2. Remove the block of tofu from the packaging. Wrap the tofu in a kitchen towel or paper towels and place a heavy object on top, like a pan or canned goods (alternatively, you can use a tofu press). Let the tofu drain for at least 15 minutes.
3. In a large mixing bowl, add about ¼ cup of cilantro, 3 tablespoons rice vinegar, 2 tablespoons toasted sesame oil, minced garlic, crushed red pepper flakes, and Swerve; whisk together.
4. Peel and julienne the eggplant. You can julienne roughly by hand, or you can use a mandolin with a julienne attachment to cut the eggplant into thin noodles.
5. Add the eggplant into bowl with marinade; toss to coat.
6. Place a skillet over medium-low heat and add olive oil. Once the oil is heated, add the eggplant and cook until it softens.

7. The eggplant will soak up all the liquids, so if you have issues with it sticking to the pan, feel free to add a little more sesame or olive oil. Just be sure to adjust your nutrition tracking.
8. Turn the oven off. Add the remaining cilantro into the eggplant then place the noodles in an oven safe dish. Cover with a lid or foil and place into the oven to keep warm.
9. Pour off fat from skillet then wipe skillet clean with paper towels. Place it back on the stovetop to heat up again.
10. Unwrap the tofu then cut into 8 slices. Spread sesame seeds over a large plate. Press both sides of each tofu slice into the sesame seeds to coat evenly. Transfer to a plate.
11. Pour 2 tablespoons of sesame oil into the skillet.
12. Arrange the tofu slices in a single layer in the skillet and cook on medium-low for about 5 minutes or until they start to crisp. With a spatula, carefully turn them over and cook for about 5 minutes on the other side.

13. Pour ¼ cup of soy sauce into the pan and coat the pieces of tofu.
14. Cook until the tofu slices look browned and caramelized with the soy sauce.
15. To serve, remove the eggplant noodles from the oven, divide them among plates and place the tofu on top.

Nutritions:

Calories: 293, Total Fats: 24.4g, Carbohydrates: 12.2g, Fiber: 5.3g, Protein: 11g

Rutabaga Hash Browns

Preparation Time: 20 minutes

Cooking Time: 10 minutes

Servings: 6

Ingredients:

- 1 large rutabaga (about 1 pound)
- ¼ cup finely grated Parmesan cheese
- 1½ teaspoons dried minced onion
- ¼ teaspoon black pepper
- ½ teaspoon sea salt
- 3 tablespoons avocado oil (or your preferred high-heat tolerant oil)

Directions:

1. Peel the outer skin from the rutabaga.
2. Chop into about 8 equal pieces.
3. Bring a medium pot of salted water to a boil.
4. Add peeled & chopped rutabaga and cook over medium-high heat for 10 minutes.

5. Place the rutabaga pieces in a colander or strainer and rinse them under cold running water then pat dry with a few paper towels.
6. Shred the rutabaga with either a grater or a food processor equipped with a shredding blade.
7. Add Parmesan cheese and minced onion to shredded rutabaga, season with salt and pepper, and mix to combine.
8. Place a large frying pan over medium-low heat and add about 1 tablespoon of oil. Once the oil is heated, add shredded rutabaga, and cook, working in batches, until crisp and golden brown on one side, 3 to 4 minutes.
9. If desired, gently press the layer down with a spatula. Then use a spatula to flip the rutabaga. Continue to cook until they are golden brown on the bottom, about 3 minutes.
10. Serve immediately.

Nutritions:

Calories: 114, Total Fats: 8g, Carbohydrates: 7g, Fiber: 2g, Protein: 3g

Crispy Flaxseed Waffles (ovo)

Preparation Time: 15 minutes

Cooking Time: 20 minutes

Servings: 8

Ingredients:

- 2 cups golden flaxseed (if available, use golden flaxseed meal)
- 5 large organic eggs (for vegan waffles, replace with 5 flax eggs)
- 1 tbsp. baking powder
- ½ cup water (slightly more if necessary)
- ⅓ cup extra virgin olive oil
- 1 tbsp. ground cinnamon
- 1 tbsp. pure vanilla extract
- 6-12 drops stevia sweetener (or more depending on desired sweetness)
- Pinch of salt
- Optional: ¼ cup toasted coconut flakes

Directions:

1. Preheat a waffle maker. If you don't have a waffle maker, heat a medium-sized skillet over medium-high heat for crispy flaxseed pancakes. Grease the waffle maker or skillet with a pinch of olive oil.
2. Take a medium-sized bowl and combine the flaxseed (or flaxseed meal) with the baking powder, eggs, water, remaining olive oil, and a pinch of salt. Incorporate all ingredients by using a whisk and allow the mixture to sit for 5 minutes.
3. Transfer the mixture to a blender or food processor and blend until foamy.
4. Pour the mixture back into the bowl and allow it to sit for another 3 minutes.
5. Add the remaining dry ingredients—except the optional toasted coconut flakes—and incorporate everything by using a whisk.
6. Scoop ¼ of the mixture into the waffle maker or skillet. Cook until a firm waffle or pancake has formed. When using a skillet, carefully flip the pancake.

7. Repeat this process for the 3 remaining parts of the batter.
8. Serve the waffles (or pancakes) with the optional toasted coconut flakes and enjoy!
9. Alternatively, store the waffles in an airtight container, keep them in the fridge, and consume within 3 days. Store for a maximum of 30 days in the freezer and thaw at room temperature.

Nutritions:

Calories: 204kcal, Net Carbs: 1.5g, Fat: 18g, Protein: 8g, Fiber: 5.9g, Sugar: 0.3g

Baked Cauliflower

Preparation Time: 15 minutes

Cooking Time: 40 minutes

Servings: 2

Ingredients:

- 1/2 cauliflower head, cut into florets
- 2 tbsp olive oil

For seasoning:

- 1/2 tsp garlic powder
- 1/2 tsp ground cumin
- 1/2 tsp black pepper
- 1 tsp onion powder
- 1/2 tsp white pepper
- 1/4 tsp dried oregano
- 1/4 tsp dried basil
- 1/4 tsp dried thyme
- 1 tbsp ground cayenne pepper
- 2 tbsp ground paprika
- 2 tsp salt

Directions:

1. Preheat the oven to 400 F/ 200 C.
2. Spray a baking tray with cooking spray and set aside.
3. In a large bowl, mix together all seasoning ingredients.
4. Add oil and stir well. Add cauliflower to the bowl seasoning mixture and stir well to coat.
5. Spread the cauliflower florets on a baking tray and bake in preheated oven for 45 minutes.
6. Serve and enjoy.

Nutritions:

Calories 177, Fat 15.6g, Carbohydrates 11.5g, Sugar 3.2g, Protein 3.1g, Cholesterol 0mg

Cabbage Cucumber Salad

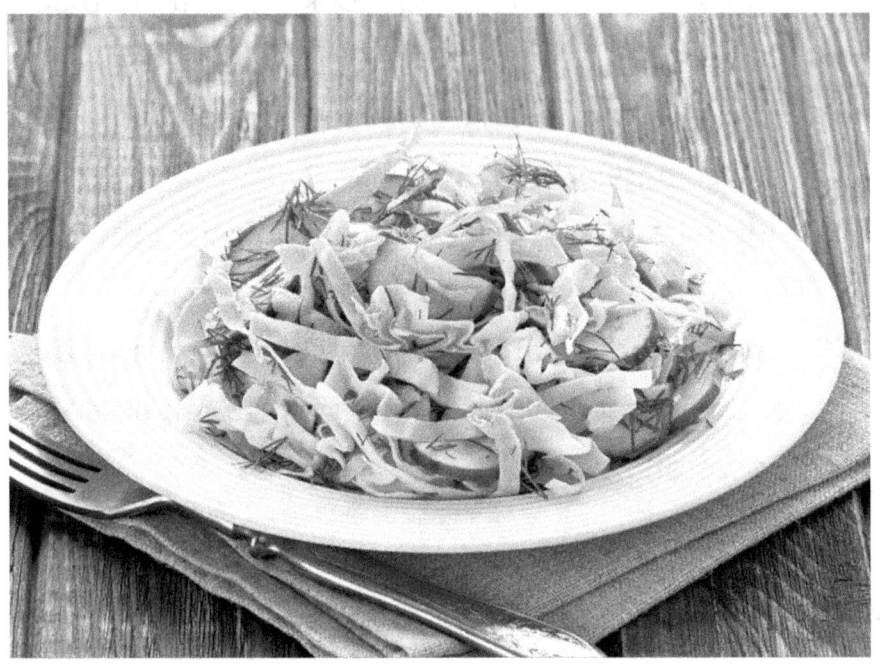

Preparation Time: 20 minutes

Cooking Time: 0 minute

Servings: 8

Ingredients:

- 1/2 cabbage head, chopped
- 2 tbsp green onion, chopped
- 2 cucumbers, sliced

- 2 tbsp fresh dill, chopped
- 3 tbsp olive oil
- 1/2 lemon juice
- Pepper
- Salt

Directions:

1. Add cabbage to the large bowl. Season with 1 teaspoon of salt mix well and set aside.
2. Add cucumbers, green onions, and fresh dill. Mix well.
3. Add lemon juice, pepper, olive oil, and salt. Mix well.
4. Place salad bowl in the refrigerator for 2 hours.
5. Serve chilled and enjoy.

Nutritions:

Calories 71, Fat 5.4g, Carbohydrates 5.9g, Sugar 2.8g, Protein 1.3g, Cholesterol 0mg

Cashew-Chocolate Truffles

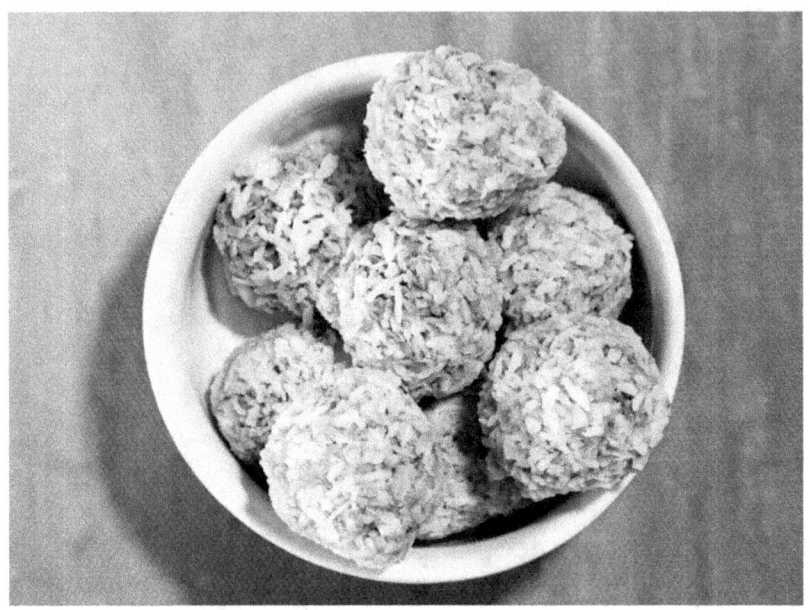

Preparation time: 15 minutes

cooking time: 0 minutes • plus 1 hour to set

servings: 12 truffles

Ingredients

- ¾ cup pitted dates
- 1 cup raw cashews, soaked in water overnight
- 2 tablespoons coconut oil
- 1 cup unsweetened shredded coconut, divided

- 1 to 2 tablespoons cocoa powder, to taste

Directions

1. In a food processor, combine the cashews, dates, coconut oil, ½ cup of shredded coconut, and cocoa powder. Pulse until fully incorporated; it will resemble chunky cookie dough. Spread the remaining ½ cup of shredded coconut on a plate.
2. Form the mixture into tablespoon-size balls and roll on the plate to cover with the shredded coconut. Transfer to a parchment paper–lined plate or baking sheet. Repeat to make 12 truffles.
3. Place the truffles in the refrigerator for 1 hour to set. Transfer the truffles to a storage container or freezer-safe bag and seal.

Nutrition (1 truffle):

Calories 238: Fat: 18g; Protein: 3g; Carbohydrates: 16g; Fiber: 4g; Sugar: 9g; Sodium: 9mg

Fruits Stew

Preparation time: 10 minutes

Cooking time: 10 minutes

Servings: 4

Ingredients:

- 1 avocado, peeled, pitted and sliced
- 1 cup plums, stoned and halved
- 2 teaspoons vanilla extract
- 1 tablespoon lemon juice
- 2 cups water
- 2 tablespoons stevia

Directions:

1. In a pan, combine the avocado with the plums, water and the other ingredients, bring to a simmer and cook over medium heat for 10 minutes.
2. Divide the mix into bowls and serve cold.

Nutrition:

calories 178, fat 4.4, fiber 2, carbs 3, protein 5

Mint Chocolate Cream

Preparation time: 10 minutes

Cooking time: 0 minutes

Servings: 6

Ingredients:

- 1 cup coconut oil, melted
- 4 tablespoons cocoa powder
- 1 cup mint, chopped
- 2 cups coconut cream
- 1 teaspoon vanilla extract
- 4 tablespoons stevia

Directions:

1. In your food processor, combine the coconut oil with the cocoa powder, the cream and the other ingredients, pulse well, divide into bowls and serve really cold.

Nutrition:

calories 514, fat 56, fiber 3.9, carbs 7.8, protein 3

Cranberries Cake

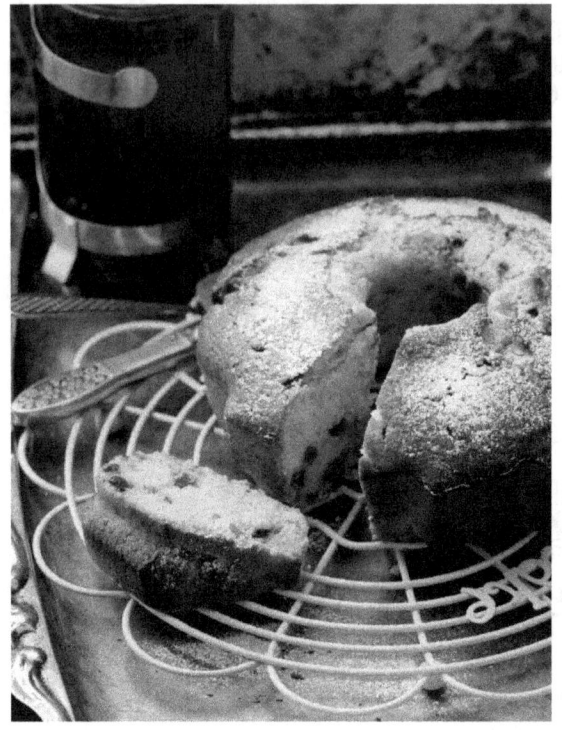

Preparation time: 10 minutes

Cooking time: 30 minutes

Servings: 6

Ingredients:

- 1 cup cranberries
- 2 cups coconut flour

- 2 tablespoon coconut oil, melted
- 1 tablespoon cocoa powder, unsweetened
- 3 tablespoons stevia
- 2 tablespoons flaxseed mixed with 3 tablespoons water
- 1 cup coconut cream
- ¼ teaspoon vanilla extract
- ½ teaspoon baking powder

Directions:

1. In a bowl, combine the coconut flour with the coconut oil, the stevia and the other ingredients, and whisk well.
2. Pour this into a cake pan lined with parchment paper, introduce in the oven and cook at 360 degrees F for 30 minutes.
3. Cool down, slice and serve.

Nutrition:

calories 244, fat 16.7, fiber 11.8, carbs 21.3, protein 4.4

Custard Bread Pudding.

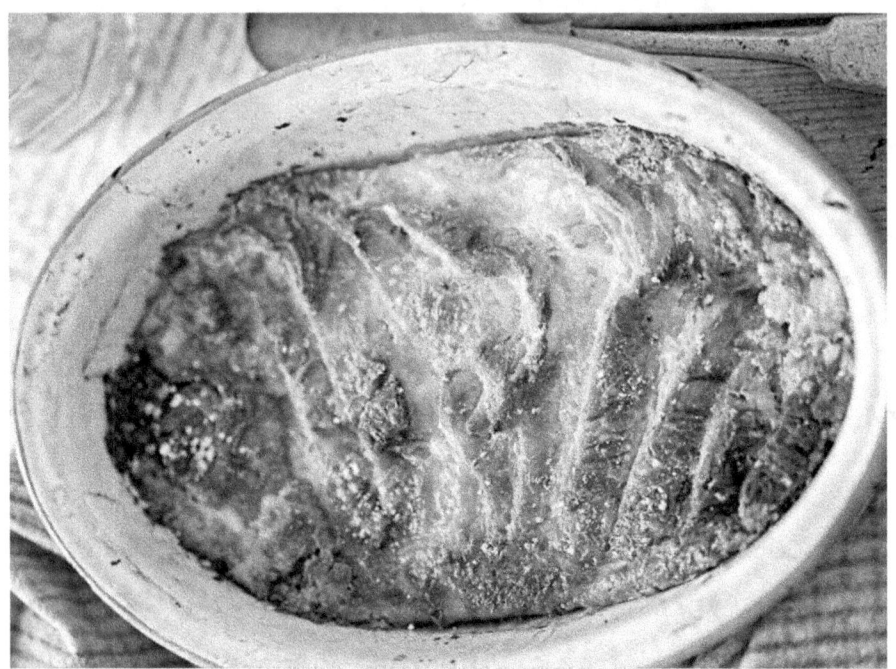

Preparation Time: 45 Minutes

Servings: 6

Ingredients:

- 6 cups cubed white bread
- 3 cups unsweetened almond milk
- 2 cups fresh raspberries or sliced strawberries, for serving

- ½ cup packed light brown sugar or granulated natural sugar
- ½ cup vegan white chocolate chips
- ½ cup dry Marsala
- Pinch of salt

Directions:

1. Melt your white chocolate into a cup of the almond milk. If using your Cooker, keep the lid off, stir throughout.
2. Add the Marsala, sugar, and salt.
3. Clean your Cooker.
4. Press half the bread cubes into the insert.
5. Pour half the Marsala mix on top.
6. Repeat.
7. Seal and cook on low for 35 minutes.
8. Release the pressure naturally.
9. Serve warm with fresh berries.

Low-Carb Curd Soufflé

Preparation time: 45 minutes

Ingredients:

For the soufflé:
- 5 Oz. cottage cheese
- 7 Oz. cream
- ½ cup condensed milk
- 1 pack (1 Oz.) gelatin for a dense soufflé
- 1 cup milk

Directions:
1. Fill the gelatin with milk and set aside.
2. Mix the condensed milk with the cream and bring to boil on a low heat.
3. Pour the gelatin mass into the boiled mixture and mix it, then let it cool.
4. In a mixer, have all the mass combined well with the cottage cheese for at least 10 minutes.
5. Pour it into the silicone moulds for the cupcakes and let it freeze for a couple of hours and serve.

Baked Rhubarb

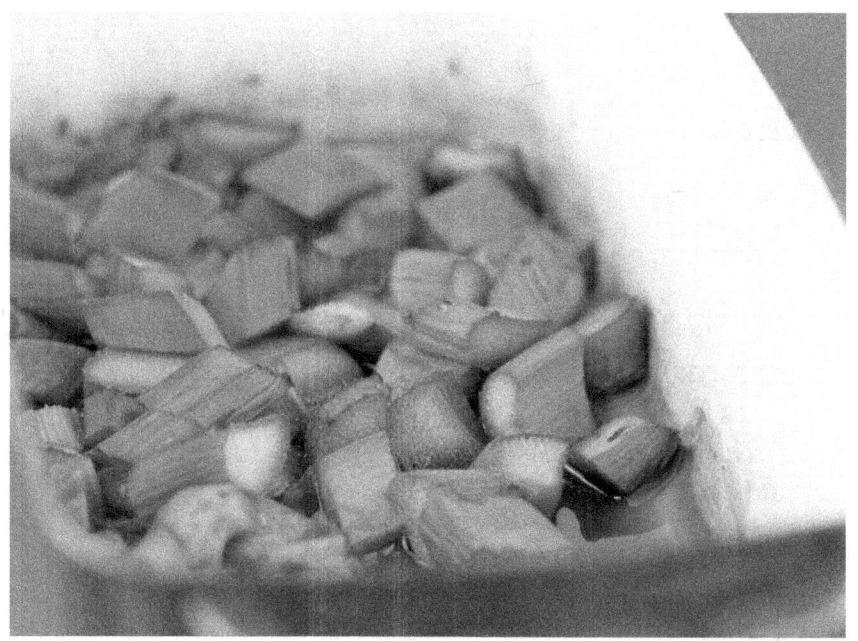

Preparation time: 10 minutes

Cooking time: 20 minutes

Servings: 4

Ingredients:

- 4 teaspoons stevia
- 1 pound rhubarb, roughly sliced
- 2 tablespoons avocado oil

- 1 teaspoon vanilla extract
- 1 teaspoon cinnamon powder
- 1 teaspoon nutmeg, ground

Directions:

1. Arrange the rhubarb on a baking sheet lined with parchment paper, add the stevia, vanilla and the other ingredients, toss and bake at 350 degrees F for 20 minutes.
2. Divide the baked rhubarb into bowls and serve cold.

Nutrition:

calories 176, fat 4.5, fiber 7.6, carbs 11.5, protein 5

Avocado Cupcakes

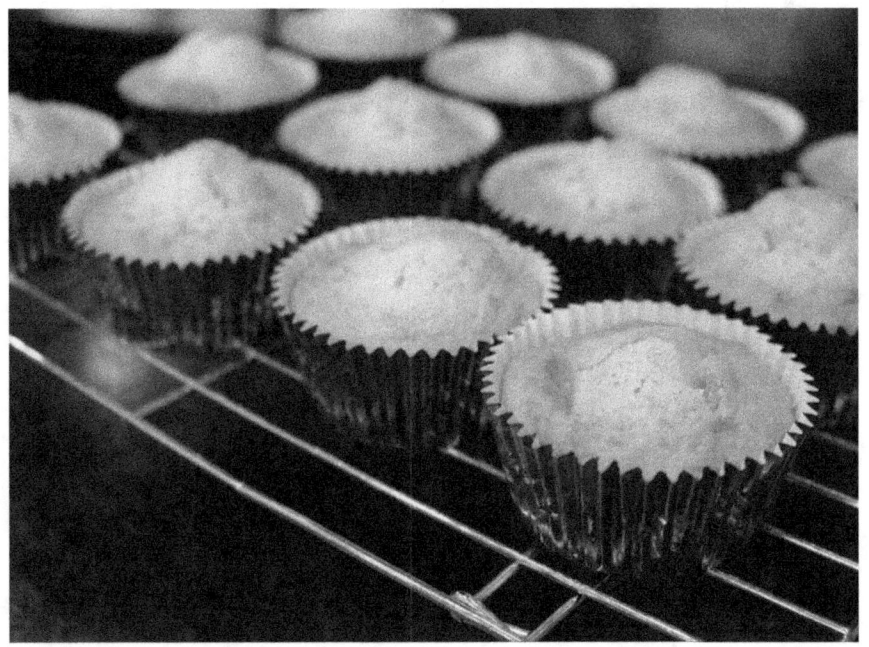

Preparation time: 10 minutes

Cooking time: 20 minutes

Servings: 4

Ingredients:

- 3 tablespoons avocado oil
- 3 tablespoons flaxseed mixed with 4 tablespoons water

- 2 teaspoons cinnamon powder
- ½ cup coconut milk
- 2 avocados, peeled, pitted and chopped
- ¾ cup coconut flour
- ½ teaspoon baking powder
- Cooking spray

Directions:

1. In a bowl, combine the avocado oil with the flaxseed mix, the milk and the other ingredients except the cooking spray, whisk well, pour in a cupcake pan greased with the cooking spray, introduce in the oven at 360 degrees F and bake for 25 minutes.
2. Cool the cupcakes down and serve.

Nutrition:

calories 142, fat 5.8, fiber 4.2, carbs 5.7, protein 1.6

Rhubarb and Berries Cream

Preparation time: 10 minutes

Cooking time: 0 minutes

Servings: 4

Ingredients:

- 2 cups rhubarb, chopped
- 1 cup blackberries
- 1 cup stevia
- 1 teaspoon vanilla extract
- 1 tablespoon avocado oil
- 1/3 cup coconut cream

Directions:

1. In a blender, combine the rhubarb with the stevia, the berries and the rest of the ingredients, pulse well, divide into cups and serve cold.

Nutrition:

calories 200, fat 5.2, fiber 3.4, carbs 7.6, protein 2.5

Chia Bowls

Preparation time: 5 minutes

Cooking time: 0 minutes

Servings: 2

Ingredients:

- 2 cups coconut milk, warm
- ½ cup coconut cream
- 2 tablespoons stevia
- 1 cup cauliflower rice, steamed
- 2 tablespoons chia seeds
- 1 teaspoon cinnamon powder

Directions:

1. In a bowl, combine the cream with the milk, the cauliflower rice and the other ingredients, whisk, well, leave aside for 5 minutes, divide into small bowls and serve cold.

Nutrition:

calories 182, fat 3.4, fiber 3.4, carbs 8.4, protein 3

Almond Butter Brownies

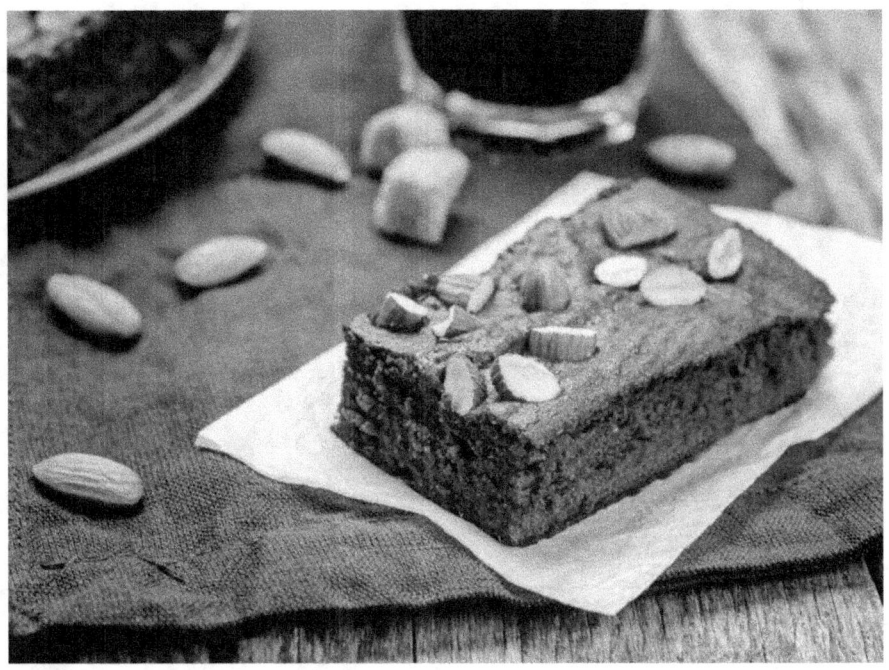

Preparation Time: 15 minutes

Cooking Time: 15 minutes

Servings: 4

Ingredients:

- 2 tbsp cocoa powder
- 1 scoop protein powder
- 1/2 cup almond butter, melted

- 1 cup bananas, overripe

Directions:

1. Preheat the oven to 350 F/ 176 C.
2. Spray brownie tray with cooking spray.
3. Add all ingredients into the blender and blend until smooth.
4. Pour batter into the prepared dish and bake in preheated oven for 20 minutes.
5. Serve and enjoy.

Nutritions:

Calories 82, Fat 2.1g, Carbohydrates 11.4g, Protein 6.9g, Sugars 5g, Cholesterol 16mg

NOTE

www.ingramcontent.com/pod-product-compliance
Lightning Source LLC
Chambersburg PA
CBHW070934080526
44589CB00013B/1514